Fatty Liver Diet Cookbook for Seniors

Dr. Mary Williams

Disclaimer

Please keep in mind that the content in this book is solely for educational purposes. The information offered here is said to be reliable and trustworthy. The author makes no implication or intends to offer any warranty of accuracy for particular individual cases.

Before beginning any diet or lifestyle habits, it is recommended that you contact a knowledgeable practitioner, such as your doctor. This book's material should not be utilized in place of expert counsel or professional guidance.

The author, publisher, and distributor expressly disclaim all liability, loss, damage, or danger incurred by persons who rely on the information in this book, whether directly or indirectly.

All intellectual property rights are retained. This book's information should not be replicated in any way, mechanically, electronically, photocopying, or by any other methods accessible

Table of Contents

Why this book is a gamechanger for seniors

Are you a senior looking to take control of your health and well-being? Do you find yourself concerned about the impact of your diet on your liver health? If the answer is yes, then you're in the right place. The "Fatty Liver Diet Cookbook for Seniors" is not just a collection of recipes; it's a comprehensive guide to transforming your lifestyle and reclaiming your health.

In our golden years, it becomes increasingly vital to prioritize our well-being, and the health of our liver is a cornerstone of overall vitality. Now, let's delve into how this cookbook can be the key to addressing your concerns.

The recipes meticulously curated within these pages are not only delicious but are specifically designed to support liver health. Each ingredient is chosen with care, focusing on their nutritional benefits and their positive impact on mitigating fatty liver issues. We understand the unique needs of seniors, and that's why this cookbook goes beyond merely providing recipes; it educates you on the science behind each ingredient and its role in promoting liver wellness.

Whether you're a novice in the kitchen or a seasoned chef, the book caters to all skill levels. The step-by-step instructions make it easy for anyone to prepare these meals, ensuring that you can effortlessly incorporate liver-friendly dishes into your daily routine.
But why is a healthy liver so crucial? Your liver plays a central role in detoxifying your body, processing nutrients, and maintaining a balanced metabolism. As we age, the liver can face challenges, and that's where this cookbook becomes your ally. By adopting the recipes and principles

outlined in this book, you're not just getting a cookbook; you're gaining a valuable resource that empowers you to make informed choices for a healthier life.

Imagine savoring meals that are not only a treat for your taste buds but also a nurturing embrace for your liver. The "Fatty Liver Diet Cookbook for Seniors" isn't just about eating; it's about making a positive change in your lifestyle that will resonate throughout your body.

So, if you're ready to embark on a journey towards improved liver health, greater vitality, and a more delicious way of living, this cookbook is your guide. Don't just eat; nourish your body with intention. Your well-being is a priority, and this cookbook is your companion on the path to a healthier and happier you.

RECIPES

Avocado and Spinach Omelette

Intro:

This nutrient-packed Avocado and Spinach Omelette is a delicious and protein-rich breakfast option. The combination of creamy avocado and vibrant spinach creates a satisfying and flavorful omelette.

Total Prep Time:

15 minutes

Ingredients:
- 2 eggs
- 1/2 avocado, diced
- 1 cup fresh spinach, chopped
- Salt and pepper to taste
- 1 tablespoon olive oil

Instructions:
1. In a bowl, whisk the eggs and season with salt and pepper.
2. Heat olive oil in a non-stick skillet over medium heat.
3. Pour the whisked eggs into the skillet, swirling to spread evenly.
4. As the edges set, add diced avocado and chopped spinach on one side of the omelette.
5. Gently fold the other half of the omelette over the filling.
6. Cook for an additional 2-3 minutes until the omelette is fully cooked but still moist inside.
7. Slide onto a plate, and enjoy!

Nutritional Information:

(Per serving)
- Calories: 320

- Protein: 18g
- Fat: 24g
- Carbohydrates: 10g
- Fiber: 6g

Quinoa Breakfast Bowl with Berries

Intro:

This Quinoa Breakfast Bowl with Berries is a wholesome and energizing way to start your day. Packed with protein from quinoa and antioxidants from fresh berries, it's a nutritious breakfast option.

Total Prep Time:

20 minutes

Ingredients:

- 1 cup cooked quinoa
- 1/2 cup mixed berries (strawberries, blueberries, raspberries)
- 1 tablespoon honey
- 1/4 cup chopped nuts (almonds, walnuts)
- 1/2 cup Greek yogurt

Instructions:

1. In a bowl, layer cooked quinoa.
2. Top with mixed berries and chopped nuts.
3. Drizzle honey over the bowl.
4. Add a dollop of Greek yogurt on top.
5. Mix well before enjoying.

Nutritional Information:

(Per serving)

- Calories: 350
- Protein: 15g

- Fat: 10g
- Carbohydrates: 50g
- Fiber: 8g

Greek Yogurt Parfait with Walnuts and Honey

Intro:
Indulge in a Greek Yogurt Parfait with Walnuts and Honey, a delightful combination of creamy yogurt, crunchy walnuts, and sweet honey. This parfait is a quick and nutritious breakfast or snack.

Total Prep Time:
10 minutes

Ingredients:
- 1 cup Greek yogurt
- 1/4 cup chopped walnuts
- 2 tablespoons honey
- 1/2 cup mixed berries

Instructions:
1. In a glass, layer Greek yogurt.
2. Add a layer of mixed berries.
3. Sprinkle chopped walnuts over the berries.
4. Drizzle honey on top.
5. Repeat the layers.
6. Finish with a dollop of Greek yogurt, a few berries, and a final drizzle of honey.

Nutritional Information:
(Per serving)
- Calories: 280
- Protein: 20g
- Fat: 15g

- Carbohydrates: 25g
- Fiber: 4g

Chia Seed Pudding with Almond Milk

Intro:
Chia Seed Pudding with Almond Milk is a nutritious and versatile breakfast option. Packed with omega-3 fatty acids and fiber, this pudding is not only delicious but also a great way to kickstart your day.

Total Prep Time:
5 minutes (plus overnight chilling)

Ingredients:
- 2 tablespoons chia seeds
- 1 cup almond milk
- 1 tablespoon maple syrup
- 1/2 teaspoon vanilla extract
- Fresh fruit for topping

Instructions:
1. In a bowl, mix chia seeds, almond milk, maple syrup, and vanilla extract.
2. Stir well and let it sit for a few minutes.
3. Stir again to prevent clumping, then cover and refrigerate overnight.
4. In the morning, give the pudding a good stir.
5. Top with fresh fruit before serving.

Nutritional Information:
(Per serving)
- Calories: 180
- Protein: 4g
- Fat: 9g

- Carbohydrates: 20g
- Fiber: 10g

Whole Grain Pancakes with Fresh Fruit

Intro:
Start your day with a stack of Whole Grain Pancakes with Fresh Fruit. These hearty pancakes are made with whole grain flour, providing a satisfying and wholesome breakfast that's both delicious and nutritious.

Total Prep Time:
25 minutes

Ingredients:
- 1 cup whole wheat flour
- 1 tablespoon baking powder
- 1 tablespoon honey
- 1 cup almond milk
- 1 egg
- Fresh fruit for topping

Instructions:
1. In a bowl, whisk together whole wheat flour, baking powder, honey, almond milk, and egg.
2. Heat a griddle or non-stick skillet over medium heat.
3. Pour 1/4 cup portions of batter onto the griddle.
4. Cook until bubbles form on the surface, then flip and cook the other side.
5. Stack the pancakes and top with fresh fruit.

Nutritional Information:
(Per serving)
- Calories: 280
- Protein: 9g

- Fat: 5g
- Carbohydrates: 50g
- Fiber: 7g

Smoked Salmon and Cream Cheese Bagel

Intro:

Elevate your breakfast with a classic Smoked Salmon and Cream Cheese Bagel. The combination of smoked salmon, creamy cheese, and a chewy bagel creates a delightful and satisfying morning treat.

Total Prep Time:

10 minutes

Ingredients:
- 1 whole grain bagel, sliced and toasted
- 2 oz smoked salmon
- 2 tablespoons cream cheese
- Capers and red onion slices for garnish

Instructions:
1. Spread cream cheese on the toasted bagel halves.
2. Arrange smoked salmon on top of the cream cheese.
3. Garnish with capers and red onion slices.
4. Serve open-faced or as a sandwich.

Nutritional Information:

(Per serving)
- Calories: 320
- Protein: 18g
- Fat: 12g
- Carbohydrates: 35g
- Fiber: 5g

Vegetable Frittata with Sweet Potatoes

Intro:

Indulge in a flavorful and hearty Vegetable Frittata with Sweet Potatoes. Packed with colorful veggies and the sweetness of sweet potatoes, this frittata is a wholesome breakfast that's both satisfying and nutritious.

Total Prep Time:

30 minutes

Ingredients:
- 4 large eggs
- 1 sweet potato, peeled and diced
- 1 bell pepper, diced
- 1 cup cherry tomatoes, halved
- 1/2 cup spinach, chopped
- 1/4 cup feta cheese, crumbled
- Salt and pepper to taste
- 1 tablespoon olive oil

Instructions:
1. Preheat the oven to 375°F (190°C).
2. In an oven-safe skillet, heat olive oil over medium heat.
3. Add sweet potatoes and cook until slightly tender.
4. Add bell pepper, cherry tomatoes, and spinach. Sauté until vegetables are softened.
5. In a bowl, whisk eggs and season with salt and pepper.
6. Pour the eggs over the vegetables in the skillet.
7. Sprinkle crumbled feta cheese on top.
8. Transfer the skillet to the preheated oven and bake for 15-20 minutes or until the frittata is set.
9. Slice and serve.

Nutritional Information:

(Per serving)

- Calories: 240
- Protein: 12g
- Fat: 14g
- Carbohydrates: 18g
- Fiber: 4g

Oatmeal with Sliced Almonds and Blueberries

Intro:

A comforting bowl of Oatmeal with Sliced Almonds and Blueberries is a nutritious and heartwarming way to start your day. Packed with fiber and antioxidants, this oatmeal is both delicious and good for you.

Total Prep Time:

10 minutes

Ingredients:

- 1/2 cup old-fashioned oats
- 1 cup almond milk
- 1/4 cup sliced almonds
- 1/2 cup fresh blueberries
- 1 tablespoon honey

Instructions:

1. In a saucepan, bring almond milk to a simmer.
2. Stir in old-fashioned oats and cook until the oats are tender.
3. Transfer the oatmeal to a bowl.
4. Top with sliced almonds and fresh blueberries.
5. Drizzle honey over the top.
6. Stir gently and enjoy.

Nutritional Information:

(Per serving)

- Calories: 280
- Protein: 8g
- Fat: 12g
- Carbohydrates: 35g
- Fiber: 7g

Cottage Cheese and Pineapple Bowl

Intro:

Experience a delightful combination of sweetness and creaminess with the Cottage Cheese and Pineapple Bowl. Packed with protein and tropical flavor, this bowl is a quick and satisfying breakfast or snack.

Total Prep Time:

5 minutes

Ingredients:

- 1 cup low-fat cottage cheese
- 1 cup fresh pineapple, diced
- 1/4 cup shredded coconut (optional)
- Mint leaves for garnish

Instructions:

1. In a bowl, scoop cottage cheese.
2. Top with diced pineapple.
3. Sprinkle shredded coconut on top if desired.
4. Garnish with mint leaves.
5. Mix gently before enjoying.

Nutritional Information:

(Per serving)

- Calories: 220

- Protein: 22g
- Fat: 5g
- Carbohydrates: 25g
- Fiber: 3g

Sweet Potato and Black Bean Breakfast Burrito

Intro:
Spice up your morning with a Sweet Potato and Black Bean Breakfast Burrito. Packed with protein, fiber, and a hint of sweetness, this burrito is a flavorful and satisfying way to start your day.

Total Prep Time:
25 minutes

Ingredients:
- 1 large sweet potato, peeled and diced
- 1 can (15 oz) black beans, drained and rinsed
- 4 large whole wheat tortillas
- 4 eggs, scrambled
- Salsa and avocado for topping
- Salt, pepper, and cumin to taste
- 1 tablespoon olive oil

Instructions:
1. In a skillet, heat olive oil over medium heat.
2. Add diced sweet potatoes and cook until tender.
3. Add black beans and season with salt, pepper, and cumin.
4. In a separate pan, scramble the eggs.
5. Warm the tortillas and assemble the burritos with sweet potato and black bean mixture, scrambled eggs, salsa, and avocado.

6. Roll the burritos and serve.

Nutritional Information:
(Per serving)
- Calories: 380
- Protein: 15g
- Fat: 12g
- Carbohydrates: 55g
- Fiber: 10g

Almond Butter Toast with Banana Slices

Intro:
Almond Butter Toast with Banana Slices is a simple yet satisfying breakfast option. Creamy almond butter paired with sweet banana slices on whole grain toast creates a delightful combination of flavors and textures.

Total Prep Time:
5 minutes

Ingredients:
- 2 slices whole grain bread, toasted
- 2 tablespoons almond butter
- 1 banana, sliced

Instructions:
1. Spread almond butter evenly on each slice of toasted bread.
2. Arrange banana slices on top of the almond butter.
3. Optionally, drizzle with honey for added sweetness.
4. Serve and enjoy this quick and nutritious breakfast.

Nutritional Information:
(Per serving)
- Calories: 280

- Protein: 8g
- Fat: 12g
- Carbohydrates: 35g
- Fiber: 7g

Veggie and Egg Muffins

Intro:
Veggie and Egg Muffins are a convenient and protein-packed breakfast option. These savory muffins are loaded with colorful vegetables and protein-rich eggs, making them perfect for a quick and nutritious morning meal.

Total Prep Time:
25 minutes

Ingredients:
- 6 eggs
- 1/2 cup bell peppers, diced
- 1/2 cup cherry tomatoes, diced
- 1/4 cup red onion, finely chopped
- 1/4 cup spinach, chopped
- Salt and pepper to taste

Instructions:
1. Preheat the oven to 350°F (175°C) and grease a muffin tin.
2. In a bowl, whisk eggs and season with salt and pepper.
3. Stir in diced vegetables.
4. Pour the egg and vegetable mixture into the muffin cups.
5. Bake for 15-20 minutes or until the muffins are set.
6. Allow to cool slightly before serving.

Nutritional Information:
(Per serving, 2 muffins)
- Calories: 180
- Protein: 12g
- Fat: 10g
- Carbohydrates: 10g
- Fiber: 2g

Berry Smoothie with Flaxseeds

Intro:
Start your day with a refreshing and nutrient-packed Berry Smoothie with Flaxseeds. This vibrant smoothie combines the goodness of mixed berries with the added benefits of flaxseeds for a delicious and wholesome breakfast.

Total Prep Time:
10 minutes

Ingredients:
- 1 cup mixed berries (strawberries, blueberries, raspberries)
- 1 banana
- 1 tablespoon flaxseeds
- 1 cup almond milk
- 1/2 cup Greek yogurt
- Ice cubes (optional)

Instructions:
1. In a blender, combine mixed berries, banana, flaxseeds, almond milk, and Greek yogurt.
2. Blend until smooth and creamy.
3. Add ice cubes if desired and blend again.
4. Pour into a glass and enjoy this nutritious and delicious berry smoothie.

Nutritional Information:
(Per serving)
- Calories: 220
- Protein: 10g
- Fat: 8g
- Carbohydrates: 30g
- Fiber: 7g

Brown Rice Porridge with Cinnamon

Intro:
Brown Rice Porridge with Cinnamon is a warm and comforting breakfast option. Made with nutritious brown rice and flavored with cinnamon, this porridge is a wholesome way to start your day.

Total Prep Time:
40 minutes

Ingredients:
- 1/2 cup brown rice
- 2 cups almond milk
- 1/2 teaspoon cinnamon
- 1 tablespoon honey
- Sliced almonds for topping

Instructions:
1. Rinse the brown rice and cook it in almond milk according to package instructions.
2. Once cooked, stir in cinnamon and honey.
3. Simmer for an additional 10 minutes until the porridge thickens.
4. Serve warm, topped with sliced almonds.

Nutritional Information:
(Per serving)
- Calories: 300
- Protein: 8g
- Fat: 6g
- Carbohydrates: 55g
- Fiber: 4g

Spinach and Mushroom Breakfast Wrap

Intro:
The Spinach and Mushroom Breakfast Wrap is a savory and nutrient-packed option for a quick breakfast on the go. Filled with sautéed spinach and mushrooms, this wrap is a delicious way to start your day.

Total Prep Time:
15 minutes

Ingredients:
- 1 whole wheat tortilla
- 1 cup spinach, chopped
- 1/2 cup mushrooms, sliced
- 2 eggs, scrambled
- 1/4 cup feta cheese, crumbled
- Salt and pepper to taste

Instructions:
1. In a pan, sauté spinach and mushrooms until wilted.
2. Scramble the eggs and add them to the pan.
3. Season with salt and pepper.
4. Warm the tortilla and fill it with the egg, spinach, and mushroom mixture.
5. Sprinkle crumbled feta cheese on top.

6. Roll the wrap and serve.

Nutritional Information:
(Per serving)
- Calories: 320
- Protein: 18g
- Fat: 14g
- Carbohydrates: 30g
- Fiber: 6g

Whole Wheat French Toast with Strawberries

Intro:
Whole Wheat French Toast with Strawberries is a wholesome twist on a classic breakfast favorite. Made with whole wheat bread and topped with fresh strawberries, this French toast is a delicious and nutritious start to your day.

Total Prep Time:
20 minutes

Ingredients:
- 4 slices whole wheat bread
- 2 eggs
- 1/2 cup almond milk
- 1 teaspoon vanilla extract
- 1/2 teaspoon cinnamon
- Fresh strawberries for topping

Instructions:
1. In a bowl, whisk together eggs, almond milk, vanilla extract, and cinnamon.
2. Dip each slice of bread into the egg mixture, coating both sides.

3. Cook on a griddle or skillet until golden brown on both sides.
4. Top with fresh strawberries before serving.

Nutritional Information:

(Per serving)

- Calories: 250
- Protein: 12g
- Fat: 8g
- Carbohydrates: 35g
- Fiber: 6g

Egg and Avocado Toast

Intro:

Elevate your breakfast with the simplicity of Egg and Avocado Toast. Creamy avocado and a perfectly cooked egg on whole grain toast create a satisfying and nutritious meal to kickstart your day.

Total Prep Time:

10 minutes

Ingredients:

- 2 slices whole grain bread, toasted
- 2 eggs
- 1 avocado, sliced
- Salt and pepper to taste
- Red pepper flakes for garnish (optional)

Instructions:

1. In a pan, cook the eggs to your preference (poached, fried, or scrambled).
2. While the eggs cook, toast the bread slices.
3. Spread avocado slices evenly on each toast.
4. Place the cooked eggs on top of the avocado.

5. Season with salt and pepper, and garnish with red pepper flakes if desired.
6. Serve immediately.

Nutritional Information:
(Per serving)
- Calories: 320
- Protein: 14g
- Fat: 18g
- Carbohydrates: 30g
- Fiber: 8g

Buckwheat Pancakes with Mixed Berries

Intro:
Buckwheat Pancakes with Mixed Berries offer a hearty and gluten-free alternative to traditional pancakes. Packed with the goodness of buckwheat and topped with a medley of berries, this breakfast option is both nutritious and delicious.

Total Prep Time:
30 minutes

Ingredients:
- 1 cup buckwheat flour
- 1 tablespoon baking powder
- 1 tablespoon honey
- 1 cup almond milk
- 1 egg
- Mixed berries for topping

Instructions:
1. In a bowl, whisk together buckwheat flour, baking powder, honey, almond milk, and egg.

2. Heat a griddle or non-stick skillet over medium heat.
3. Pour 1/4 cup portions of batter onto the griddle.
4. Cook until bubbles form on the surface, then flip and cook the other side.
5. Stack the pancakes and top with mixed berries.

Nutritional Information:
(Per serving)
- Calories: 280
- Protein: 10g
- Fat: 6g
- Carbohydrates: 50g
- Fiber: 8g

Breakfast Quinoa with Nuts and Dried Fruit

Intro:
Start your day with a protein-packed Breakfast Quinoa with Nuts and Dried Fruit. Quinoa is cooked to perfection and mixed with a variety of nuts and dried fruit for a flavorful and nutritious breakfast bowl.

Total Prep Time:
20 minutes

Ingredients:
- 1/2 cup quinoa, rinsed
- 1 cup almond milk
- 1/4 cup mixed nuts (almonds, walnuts, pistachios), chopped
- 2 tablespoons dried fruit (raisins, cranberries)
- 1 tablespoon honey
- 1/2 teaspoon cinnamon

Instructions:

1. In a saucepan, combine quinoa and almond milk.
2. Bring to a simmer, then reduce heat, cover, and cook until quinoa is tender.
3. Fluff the quinoa with a fork and stir in mixed nuts, dried fruit, honey, and cinnamon.
4. Mix well and serve warm.

Nutritional Information:

(Per serving)

- Calories: 320
- Protein: 12g
- Fat: 10g
- Carbohydrates: 50g
- Fiber: 6g

Greek Yogurt and Berry Smoothie Bowl

Intro:

Indulge in the goodness of a Greek Yogurt and Berry Smoothie Bowl. This vibrant and satisfying bowl is loaded with the protein of Greek yogurt and the antioxidant-rich flavors of mixed berries for a delightful breakfast experience.

Total Prep Time:

10 minutes

Ingredients:

- 1 cup Greek yogurt
- 1/2 cup mixed berries (strawberries, blueberries, raspberries)
- 1 tablespoon honey
- 1/4 cup granola
- Chia seeds for topping

Instructions:

1. In a bowl, scoop Greek yogurt.
2. Top with mixed berries.
3. Drizzle honey over the bowl.
4. Sprinkle granola and chia seeds on top.
5. Mix well before enjoying this nutritious and delicious smoothie bowl.

Nutritional Information:

(Per serving)

- Calories: 280
- Protein: 20g
- Fat: 10g
- Carbohydrates: 30g
- Fiber: 4g

Turkey and Vegetable Breakfast Skillet

Intro:

The Turkey and Vegetable Breakfast Skillet is a hearty and protein-packed way to kickstart your morning. This savory skillet combines lean turkey with a variety of colorful vegetables for a delicious and nutritious breakfast.

Total Prep Time:

20 minutes

Ingredients:

- 1/2 lb lean ground turkey
- 1 bell pepper, diced
- 1 zucchini, diced
- 1 cup cherry tomatoes, halved
- 1/2 onion, finely chopped
- 2 cloves garlic, minced
- 4 eggs

- Salt and pepper to taste
- Fresh herbs for garnish (optional)

Instructions:

1. In a skillet, cook ground turkey until browned. Set aside.
2. In the same skillet, sauté bell pepper, zucchini, cherry tomatoes, onion, and garlic until vegetables are tender.
3. Add the cooked turkey back to the skillet and mix well.
4. Create wells in the mixture and crack an egg into each well.
5. Cover and cook until eggs are done to your liking.
6. Season with salt and pepper, garnish with fresh herbs if desired, and serve.

Nutritional Information:

(Per serving)

- Calories: 320
- Protein: 25g
- Fat: 15g
- Carbohydrates: 20g
- Fiber: 5g

Whole Grain Waffles with Greek Yogurt

Intro:

Whole Grain Waffles with Greek Yogurt offer a wholesome twist on a breakfast classic. These waffles are made with whole grain flour for added fiber and topped with creamy Greek yogurt for a delicious and nutritious morning treat.

Total Prep Time:

30 minutes

Ingredients:

- 1 cup whole grain flour
- 1 tablespoon baking powder
- 1 tablespoon honey
- 1 cup almond milk
- 1 egg
- Greek yogurt for topping
- Fresh fruit for garnish

Instructions:

1. In a bowl, whisk together whole grain flour, baking powder, honey, almond milk, and egg.
2. Preheat a waffle iron and lightly grease.
3. Pour batter onto the hot waffle iron and cook according to the manufacturer's instructions.
4. Once cooked, top the waffles with a generous dollop of Greek yogurt and fresh fruit.

Nutritional Information:

(Per serving)

- Calories: 280
- Protein: 10g
- Fat: 8g
- Carbohydrates: 40g
- Fiber: 6g

Apple Cinnamon Overnight Oats

Intro:

Apple Cinnamon Overnight Oats are a convenient and delicious way to start your day. These oats are soaked overnight, allowing the flavors to meld, and are topped with fresh apples and a hint of cinnamon for a delightful breakfast.

Total Prep Time:
5 minutes (plus overnight chilling)

Ingredients:
- 1/2 cup rolled oats
- 1/2 cup almond milk
- 1/2 apple, diced
- 1 tablespoon chia seeds
- 1 tablespoon honey
- 1/2 teaspoon cinnamon

Instructions:
1. In a jar, combine rolled oats, almond milk, diced apple, chia seeds, honey, and cinnamon.
2. Stir well, ensuring oats are fully submerged in the liquid.
3. Cover and refrigerate overnight.
4. In the morning, give the oats a good stir and top with additional apple slices if desired.
5. Enjoy this nutritious and easy-to-make breakfast.

Nutritional Information:
(Per serving)
- Calories: 250
- Protein: 6g
- Fat: 8g
- Carbohydrates: 40g
- Fiber: 8g

Scrambled Tofu with Spinach and Tomatoes

Intro:
Scrambled Tofu with Spinach and Tomatoes is a protein-packed and plant-based breakfast option. Tofu is

crumbled and cooked with vibrant spinach and tomatoes for a flavorful and nutritious morning meal.

Total Prep Time:
15 minutes

Ingredients:
- 1 block firm tofu, crumbled
- 1 cup fresh spinach, chopped
- 1 cup cherry tomatoes, halved
- 1/2 onion, finely chopped
- 2 cloves garlic, minced
- 1 tablespoon nutritional yeast (optional)
- Salt and pepper to taste
- 1 tablespoon olive oil

Instructions:
1. In a pan, heat olive oil over medium heat.
2. Add onion and garlic, sautéing until fragrant.
3. Add crumbled tofu to the pan and cook until slightly golden.
4. Stir in chopped spinach and halved cherry tomatoes.
5. Continue cooking until spinach wilts and tomatoes soften.
6. Season with nutritional yeast, salt, and pepper.
7. Serve this flavorful scrambled tofu on toast or as a standalone dish.

Nutritional Information:
(Per serving)
- Calories: 280
- Protein: 20g
- Fat: 18g
- Carbohydrates: 14g

- Fiber: 4g

Banana Nut Muffins with Whole Wheat Flour

Intro:
Banana Nut Muffins with Whole Wheat Flour are a wholesome and delicious treat for breakfast. Made with ripe bananas and whole wheat flour, these muffins are loaded with flavor and provide a satisfying start to your day.

Total Prep Time:
25 minutes

Ingredients:
- 2 ripe bananas, mashed
- 1/2 cup Greek yogurt
- 1/4 cup honey
- 1 egg
- 1 teaspoon vanilla extract
- 1 cup whole wheat flour
- 1/2 teaspoon baking soda
- 1/2 teaspoon baking powder
- 1/4 teaspoon salt
- 1/2 cup chopped nuts (walnuts, pecans)

Instructions:
1. Preheat the oven to 350°F (175°C) and line a muffin tin with paper liners.
2. In a bowl, mix mashed bananas, Greek yogurt, honey, egg, and vanilla extract.
3. In a separate bowl, whisk together whole wheat flour, baking soda, baking powder, and salt.

4. Combine wet and dry ingredients, then fold in chopped nuts.
5. Spoon the batter into muffin cups and bake for 18-20 minutes or until a toothpick comes out clean.
6. Allow muffins to cool before serving.

Nutritional Information:

(Per serving, 1 muffin)

- Calories: 180
- Protein: 6g
- Fat: 8g
- Carbohydrates: 24g
- Fiber: 3g

Grilled Chicken Salad with Mixed Greens

Intro:

Indulge in the freshness of a Grilled Chicken Salad with Mixed Greens. This vibrant salad features succulent grilled chicken breast atop a bed of crisp mixed greens, offering a satisfying and healthy dining experience.

Total Prep Time:

20 minutes

Ingredients:

- 2 boneless, skinless chicken breasts
- Mixed salad greens (lettuce, spinach, arugula)
- Cherry tomatoes, halved
- Cucumber, sliced
- Red onion, thinly sliced
- Balsamic vinaigrette dressing
- Olive oil for grilling
- Salt and pepper to taste

Instructions:

1. Preheat the grill or grill pan over medium-high heat.
2. Season chicken breasts with salt and pepper.
3. Grill chicken for 6-8 minutes per side or until fully cooked.
4. In a large bowl, combine mixed greens, cherry tomatoes, cucumber, and red onion.
5. Slice grilled chicken and place it on top of the salad.
6. Drizzle with balsamic vinaigrette dressing and olive oil.
7. Toss gently and serve.

Nutritional Information:

(Per serving)

- Calories: 350
- Protein: 30g
- Fat: 15g
- Carbohydrates: 20g
- Fiber: 5g

Quinoa and Black Bean Stuffed Peppers

Intro:

Quinoa and Black Bean Stuffed Peppers are a wholesome and flavorful dish that combines the nuttiness of quinoa, the richness of black beans, and the vibrant sweetness of bell peppers.

Total Prep Time:

40 minutes

Ingredients:

- 4 bell peppers, halved and seeds removed
- 1 cup quinoa, cooked
- 1 can (15 oz) black beans, drained and rinsed

- 1 cup corn kernels
- 1 cup diced tomatoes
- 1 teaspoon cumin
- 1 teaspoon chili powder
- Salt and pepper to taste
- Shredded cheese for topping (optional)

Instructions:
1. Preheat the oven to 375°F (190°C).
2. In a bowl, mix cooked quinoa, black beans, corn, diced tomatoes, cumin, chili powder, salt, and pepper.
3. Stuff each bell pepper half with the quinoa and black bean mixture.
4. Place stuffed peppers in a baking dish and cover with aluminum foil.
5. Bake for 25-30 minutes or until peppers are tender.
6. Optionally, sprinkle shredded cheese on top and bake for an additional 5 minutes.
7. Serve these flavorful stuffed peppers warm.

Nutritional Information:
(Per serving)
- Calories: 300
- Protein: 15g
- Fat: 5g
- Carbohydrates: 50g
- Fiber: 12g

Lentil Soup with Vegetables

Intro:
Lentil Soup with Vegetables is a comforting and nutritious soup that combines the earthy flavors of lentils with a

variety of colorful vegetables, creating a hearty and wholesome meal.

Total Prep Time:

30 minutes

Ingredients:

- 1 cup dry lentils, rinsed
- 1 onion, diced
- 2 carrots, sliced
- 2 celery stalks, chopped
- 3 cloves garlic, minced
- 1 can (14 oz) diced tomatoes
- 6 cups vegetable broth
- 1 teaspoon cumin
- 1 teaspoon paprika
- Salt and pepper to taste
- Fresh parsley for garnish

Instructions:

1. In a large pot, sauté onions, carrots, celery, and garlic until softened.
2. Add lentils, diced tomatoes, vegetable broth, cumin, paprika, salt, and pepper.
3. Bring to a boil, then reduce heat and simmer for 20-25 minutes or until lentils are tender.
4. Adjust seasoning to taste.
5. Garnish with fresh parsley before serving.

Nutritional Information:

(Per serving)

- Calories: 250
- Protein: 15g
- Fat: 2g
- Carbohydrates: 45g

- Fiber: 15g

Turkey and Avocado Wrap with Whole Grain Tortilla

Intro:
The Turkey and Avocado Wrap with Whole Grain Tortilla is a balanced and satisfying lunch option. Lean turkey, creamy avocado, and crisp vegetables come together in a whole grain tortilla for a delicious and nutritious wrap.

Total Prep Time:
15 minutes

Ingredients:
- 4 whole grain tortillas
- 1/2 lb lean turkey breast, sliced
- 1 avocado, sliced
- Lettuce leaves
- Tomato, thinly sliced
- Greek yogurt or your favorite dressing
- Salt and pepper to taste

Instructions:
1. Lay out the whole grain tortillas.
2. Place sliced turkey on each tortilla.
3. Add avocado slices, lettuce leaves, and tomato slices.
4. Drizzle with Greek yogurt or your favorite dressing.
5. Season with salt and pepper.
6. Wrap tightly and secure with toothpicks if needed.
7. Serve these flavorful wraps for a quick and healthy lunch.

Nutritional Information:
(Per serving)
- Calories: 320
- Protein: 25g
- Fat: 12g
- Carbohydrates: 30g
- Fiber: 8g

Greek Salad with Salmon

Intro:
Experience the Mediterranean flavors with a Greek Salad with Salmon. This refreshing salad combines crisp cucumbers, juicy tomatoes, Kalamata olives, and feta cheese, topped with grilled salmon for a protein-rich twist.

Total Prep Time:
25 minutes

Ingredients:
- 2 salmon fillets
- Mixed salad greens
- Cucumber, sliced
- Cherry tomatoes, halved
- Kalamata olives
- Feta cheese, crumbled
- Red onion, thinly sliced
- Greek dressing
- Lemon wedges for garnish

Instructions:
1. Season salmon fillets with salt and pepper.
2. Grill salmon for 4-5 minutes per side or until cooked.

3. In a large bowl, combine mixed greens, cucumber, cherry tomatoes, Kalamata olives, feta cheese, and red onion.
4. Place grilled salmon on top of the salad.
5. Drizzle with Greek dressing and garnish with lemon wedges.
6. Toss gently and serve this delightful Greek Salad with Salmon.

Nutritional Information:

(Per serving)

- Calories: 380
- Protein: 30g
- Fat: 20g
- Carbohydrates: 18g
- Fiber: 5g

Chickpea and Vegetable Stir-Fry

Intro:

Chickpea and Vegetable Stir-Fry is a quick and flavorful dish that combines protein-packed chickpeas with a medley of colorful vegetables. This stir-fry is both satisfying and easy to customize with your favorite veggies.

Total Prep Time:

20 minutes

Ingredients:

- 1 can (15 oz) chickpeas, drained and rinsed
- Broccoli florets
- Bell peppers, sliced
- Snap peas
- Carrots, julienned
- 3 cloves garlic, minced

- 1 tablespoon ginger, grated
- Soy sauce
- Sesame oil
- Red pepper flakes (optional)
- Green onions for garnish

Instructions:
1. In a wok or skillet, heat sesame oil over medium-high heat.
2. Add garlic and ginger, sautéing until fragrant.
3. Add chickpeas, broccoli, bell peppers, snap peas, and carrots.
4. Stir-fry for 5-7 minutes or until vegetables are crisp-tender.
5. Drizzle with soy sauce and add red pepper flakes if desired.
6. Garnish with green onions before serving.

Nutritional Information:
(Per serving)
- Calories: 280
- Protein: 12g
- Fat: 8g
- Carbohydrates: 40g
- Fiber: 10g

Spinach and Quinoa Salad with Feta

Intro:
The Spinach and Quinoa Salad with Feta is a nutritious and satisfying option for a light lunch or dinner. Fresh spinach, protein-rich quinoa, cherry tomatoes, and feta cheese come together with a tangy vinaigrette for a delightful salad.

Total Prep Time:
25 minutes

Ingredients:
- 2 cups fresh spinach leaves
- 1 cup cooked quinoa, cooled
- Cherry tomatoes, halved
- Red onion, thinly sliced
- Feta cheese, crumbled
- Balsamic vinaigrette dressing
- Olive oil
- Salt and pepper to taste

Instructions:
1. In a large bowl, combine fresh spinach, cooked quinoa, cherry tomatoes, red onion, and feta cheese.
2. Drizzle with balsamic vinaigrette dressing and olive oil.
3. Season with salt and pepper.
4. Toss gently to coat the salad with the dressing.
5. Serve this Spinach and Quinoa Salad as a refreshing and nutritious meal.

Nutritional Information:
(Per serving)
- Calories: 320
- Protein: 12g
- Fat: 15g
- Carbohydrates: 40g
- Fiber: 8g

Brown Rice Bowl with Tofu and Vegetables

Intro:
The Brown Rice Bowl with Tofu and Vegetables is a wholesome and plant-based dish that combines the

goodness of brown rice, tofu, and a colorful array of vegetables. This bowl is both satisfying and nutrient-packed.

Total Prep Time:

30 minutes

Ingredients:
- 1 cup brown rice, cooked
- 1 block firm tofu, cubed
- Broccoli florets
- Carrots, sliced
- Bell peppers, sliced
- 1 tablespoon soy sauce
- 1 tablespoon sesame oil
- Garlic powder and ginger powder
- Sesame seeds for garnish
- Green onions, sliced

Instructions:
1. In a pan, heat sesame oil over medium-high heat.
2. Add cubed tofu and cook until golden on all sides.
3. Add broccoli, carrots, and bell peppers to the pan.
4. Sprinkle with garlic powder and ginger powder.
5. Drizzle with soy sauce and toss to coat.
6. In a bowl, assemble brown rice, tofu, and vegetables.
7. Garnish with sesame seeds and sliced green onions.

Nutritional Information:
(Per serving)
- Calories: 350
- Protein: 15g
- Fat: 12g
- Carbohydrates: 45g

- Fiber: 8g

Whole Wheat Pasta with Tomato and Basil Sauce

Intro:
Whole Wheat Pasta with Tomato and Basil Sauce is a simple and wholesome pasta dish that combines the richness of whole wheat pasta with the classic flavors of tomato and basil. This quick and flavorful recipe is perfect for a satisfying meal.

Total Prep Time:
20 minutes

Ingredients:
- 8 oz whole wheat pasta
- 2 cups cherry tomatoes, halved
- 2 cloves garlic, minced
- Fresh basil, chopped
- 2 tablespoons olive oil
- Salt and pepper to taste
- Grated Parmesan cheese for topping (optional)

Instructions:
1. Cook whole wheat pasta according to package instructions.
2. In a pan, heat olive oil over medium heat.
3. Add minced garlic and sauté until fragrant.
4. Add cherry tomatoes to the pan and cook until they start to burst.
5. Season with salt and pepper, and stir in fresh basil.
6. Toss cooked pasta in the sauce, ensuring it's well coated.
7. Top with grated Parmesan cheese if desired.

8. Serve this delightful Whole Wheat Pasta with Tomato and Basil Sauce.

Nutritional Information:
(Per serving)

- Calories: 350
- Protein: 10g
- Fat: 8g
- Carbohydrates: 60g
- Fiber: 8g

Tuna Salad Lettuce Wraps

Intro:
Tuna Salad Lettuce Wraps offer a light and protein-packed lunch option. This recipe combines flaky tuna with crisp vegetables, wrapped in fresh lettuce leaves for a refreshing and satisfying meal.

Total Prep Time:
15 minutes

Ingredients:

- 2 cans (5 oz each) tuna, drained
- Celery, finely chopped
- Red onion, finely chopped
- Mayonnaise
- Dijon mustard
- Salt and pepper to taste
- Lettuce leaves for wrapping

Instructions:

1. In a bowl, mix tuna, chopped celery, and red onion.
2. In a separate bowl, whisk together mayonnaise and Dijon mustard.

3. Combine the tuna mixture with the dressing.
4. Season with salt and pepper to taste.
5. Spoon the tuna salad onto lettuce leaves.
6. Wrap and secure with toothpicks if needed.
7. Enjoy these Tuna Salad Lettuce Wraps for a light and satisfying lunch.

Nutritional Information:

(Per serving)

- Calories: 250
- Protein: 20g
- Fat: 12g
- Carbohydrates: 10g
- Fiber: 2g

Sweet Potato and Chickpea Curry

Intro:

Sweet Potato and Chickpea Curry is a hearty and flavorful dish that combines the natural sweetness of sweet potatoes with the protein-rich goodness of chickpeas. This curry is a comforting and nutritious option for a wholesome dinner.

Total Prep Time:

40 minutes

Ingredients:

- 2 sweet potatoes, peeled and diced
- 1 can (15 oz) chickpeas, drained and rinsed
- 1 onion, finely chopped
- 2 cloves garlic, minced
- 1 can (14 oz) diced tomatoes
- 1 can (14 oz) coconut milk
- 2 tablespoons curry powder
- 1 teaspoon turmeric

- Salt and pepper to taste
- Fresh cilantro for garnish

Instructions:

1. In a pot, sauté chopped onion and garlic until softened.
2. Add diced sweet potatoes, chickpeas, diced tomatoes, coconut milk, curry powder, turmeric, salt, and pepper.
3. Bring to a simmer and cook until sweet potatoes are tender.
4. Adjust seasoning to taste.
5. Garnish with fresh cilantro before serving.

Nutritional Information:

(Per serving)

- Calories: 380
- Protein: 10g
- Fat: 15g
- Carbohydrates: 55g
- Fiber: 12g

Caprese Sandwich with Whole Grain Bread

Intro:

Caprese Sandwich with Whole Grain Bread is a delightful and wholesome lunch option. Fresh tomatoes, mozzarella, and basil are layered on whole grain bread, drizzled with balsamic glaze, creating a flavorful and satisfying sandwich.

Total Prep Time:

15 minutes

Ingredients:

- Whole grain bread slices

- Fresh tomatoes, sliced
- Fresh mozzarella, sliced
- Fresh basil leaves
- Balsamic glaze
- Olive oil
- Salt and pepper to taste

Instructions:
1. Arrange whole grain bread slices on a clean surface.
2. Layer sliced tomatoes, mozzarella, and fresh basil on half of the bread slices.
3. Drizzle with balsamic glaze and olive oil.
4. Season with salt and pepper.
5. Top with the remaining bread slices to create sandwiches.
6. Slice in half and serve these Caprese Sandwiches for a light and tasty lunch.

Nutritional Information:
(Per serving)
- Calories: 280
- Protein: 12g
- Fat: 10g
- Carbohydrates: 35g
- Fiber: 6g

Shrimp and Vegetable Skewers

Intro:
Shrimp and Vegetable Skewers are a quick and flavorful option for a light dinner or outdoor barbecue. Succulent shrimp, colorful vegetables, and a zesty marinade come together for a delicious and healthy meal.

Total Prep Time:
30 minutes

Ingredients:
- Shrimp, peeled and deveined
- Cherry tomatoes
- Bell peppers, cut into chunks
- Zucchini, sliced
- Red onion, cut into wedges
- Olive oil
- Garlic, minced
- Lemon juice
- Paprika, cumin, and oregano
- Salt and pepper to taste

Instructions:
1. In a bowl, mix olive oil, minced garlic, lemon juice, paprika, cumin, oregano, salt, and pepper to create a marinade.
2. Thread shrimp, cherry tomatoes, bell peppers, zucchini, and red onion onto skewers.
3. Brush the skewers with the marinade.
4. Grill or bake until shrimp are opaque and vegetables are tender.
5. Serve these Shrimp and Vegetable Skewers as a flavorful and light dinner.

Nutritional Information:
(Per serving)
- Calories: 250
- Protein: 20g
- Fat: 12g
- Carbohydrates: 15g
- Fiber: 4g

Minestrone Soup with Whole Grain Pasta

Intro:

Minestrone Soup with Whole Grain Pasta is a hearty and comforting soup that combines a medley of vegetables, beans, and whole grain pasta in a flavorful broth. This classic Italian soup is wholesome and satisfying.

Total Prep Time:

45 minutes

Ingredients:

- 1 cup whole grain pasta, cooked
- 1 onion, diced
- 2 carrots, sliced
- 2 celery stalks, chopped
- 3 cloves garlic, minced
- 1 can (14 oz) diced tomatoes
- 1 can (15 oz) kidney beans, drained and rinsed
- 6 cups vegetable broth
- 1 teaspoon dried oregano
- 1 teaspoon dried basil
- Salt and pepper to taste
- Parmesan cheese for topping (optional)

Instructions:

1. In a large pot, sauté diced onion, sliced carrots, chopped celery, and minced garlic until softened.
2. Add diced tomatoes, kidney beans, vegetable broth, dried oregano, dried basil, salt, and pepper.
3. Simmer for 30 minutes.
4. Stir in cooked whole grain pasta.
5. Adjust seasoning to taste.
6. Serve this Minestrone Soup hot, optionally topped with Parmesan cheese.

Nutritional Information:
(Per serving)
- Calories: 300
- Protein: 12g
- Fat: 4g
- Carbohydrates: 55g
- Fiber: 10g

Chicken and Vegetable Quinoa Bowl

Intro:
The Chicken and Vegetable Quinoa Bowl is a balanced and protein-packed meal that combines tender chicken, colorful vegetables, and fluffy quinoa. This bowl is both nutritious and satisfying, making it a perfect lunch or dinner option.

Total Prep Time:
25 minutes

Ingredients:
- 1 cup quinoa, cooked
- Boneless, skinless chicken breast, sliced
- Broccoli florets
- Bell peppers, sliced
- Cherry tomatoes, halved
- Olive oil
- Garlic powder, paprika, and cumin
- Salt and pepper to taste
- Lemon wedges for garnish

Instructions:
1. In a pan, heat olive oil over medium-high heat.
2. Season sliced chicken with garlic powder, paprika, cumin, salt, and pepper.

3. Cook chicken until browned and cooked through.
4. In the same pan, sauté broccoli, bell peppers, and cherry tomatoes until tender.
5. In a bowl, assemble cooked quinoa, chicken, and sautéed vegetables.
6. Garnish with lemon wedges before serving.

Nutritional Information:

(Per serving)

- Calories: 380
- Protein: 30g
- Fat: 15g
- Carbohydrates: 35g
- Fiber: 6g

Black Bean and Corn Salad

Intro:

Black Bean and Corn Salad is a refreshing and nutritious side dish that combines black beans, sweet corn, crisp vegetables, and a zesty dressing. This salad is versatile and can be served on its own or as a topping for tacos or grilled meats.

Total Prep Time:

15 minutes

Ingredients:

- 1 can (15 oz) black beans, drained and rinsed
- 1 cup corn kernels (fresh or frozen)
- Red bell pepper, diced
- Red onion, finely chopped
- Fresh cilantro, chopped
- Lime juice
- Olive oil

- Cumin, chili powder, and salt to taste
- Avocado slices for garnish

Instructions:

1. In a bowl, combine black beans, corn, diced red bell pepper, and finely chopped red onion.
2. In a small bowl, whisk together lime juice, olive oil, cumin, chili powder, and salt to create the dressing.
3. Pour the dressing over the bean and corn mixture.
4. Add fresh cilantro and toss gently to combine.
5. Garnish with avocado slices before serving.

Nutritional Information:

(Per serving)

- Calories: 250
- Protein: 10g
- Fat: 8g
- Carbohydrates: 40g
- Fiber: 10g

Turkey and Vegetable Lettuce Wraps

Intro:

Turkey and Vegetable Lettuce Wraps are a light and flavorful alternative to traditional wraps. Ground turkey is seasoned and sautéed with crisp vegetables, then wrapped in fresh lettuce leaves for a nutritious and low-carb meal.

Total Prep Time:

20 minutes

Ingredients:

- 1 lb lean ground turkey
- Lettuce leaves (butter lettuce or iceberg)
- Bell peppers, diced

- Carrots, julienned
- Green onions, sliced
- Soy sauce, hoisin sauce, and sesame oil
- Garlic powder and ginger powder
- Sesame seeds for garnish

Instructions:
1. In a pan, cook ground turkey until browned.
2. Add diced bell peppers, julienned carrots, and sliced green onions.
3. In a small bowl, mix soy sauce, hoisin sauce, sesame oil, garlic powder, and ginger powder.
4. Pour the sauce over the turkey and vegetable mixture.
5. Stir well and cook until vegetables are tender.
6. Spoon the turkey mixture onto lettuce leaves.
7. Sprinkle with sesame seeds for garnish.
8. Enjoy these Turkey and Vegetable Lettuce Wraps for a light and flavorful meal.

Nutritional Information:
(Per serving)
- Calories: 280
- Protein: 25g
- Fat: 12g
- Carbohydrates: 15g
- Fiber: 5g

Whole Wheat Pita with Hummus and Veggies

Intro:
Whole Wheat Pita with Hummus and Veggies is a satisfying and nutritious snack or light lunch. Whole wheat

pita is filled with creamy hummus and an assortment of fresh vegetables for a flavorful and wholesome treat.

Total Prep Time:

10 minutes

Ingredients:
- Whole wheat pitas
- Hummus (store-bought or homemade)
- Cherry tomatoes, halved
- Cucumber, sliced
- Bell peppers, sliced
- Baby carrots
- Kalamata olives, pitted
- Fresh parsley, chopped

Instructions:
1. Warm whole wheat pitas in a toaster or microwave.
2. Spread a generous layer of hummus on each pita.
3. Arrange cherry tomatoes, cucumber slices, bell pepper slices, baby carrots, and Kalamata olives on top.
4. Sprinkle with fresh parsley for added flavor.
5. Fold the pita in half and enjoy this Whole Wheat Pita with Hummus and Veggies as a nutritious snack.

Nutritional Information:

(Per serving)
- Calories: 280
- Protein: 8g
- Fat: 10g
- Carbohydrates: 40g
- Fiber: 8g

Salmon and Asparagus Quiche

Intro:

Salmon and Asparagus Quiche is an elegant and flavorful dish that combines the richness of salmon, the freshness of asparagus, and the creaminess of eggs and cheese. This quiche is perfect for brunch or a light dinner.

Total Prep Time:

40 minutes

Ingredients:
- Pie crust (store-bought or homemade)
- Smoked salmon, flaked
- Asparagus spears, trimmed and blanched
- Eggs
- Milk or cream
- Swiss cheese, grated
- Dill, chopped
- Salt and pepper to taste

Instructions:
1. Preheat the oven to 375°F (190°C).
2. Roll out the pie crust and line a pie dish.
3. Arrange flaked smoked salmon and blanched asparagus in the crust.
4. In a bowl, whisk together eggs, milk or cream, grated Swiss cheese, chopped dill, salt, and pepper.
5. Pour the egg mixture over the salmon and asparagus.
6. Bake for 25-30 minutes or until the quiche is set and golden brown.
7. Allow to cool slightly before slicing.
8. Serve this delightful Salmon and Asparagus Quiche for a sophisticated meal.

Nutritional Information:
(Per serving)

- Calories: 320
- Protein: 18g
- Fat: 22g
- Carbohydrates: 15g
- Fiber: 2g

Quinoa and Kale Stuffed Tomatoes

Intro:

Quinoa and Kale Stuffed Tomatoes are a wholesome and colorful dish that brings together the nuttiness of quinoa, the earthiness of kale, and the freshness of ripe tomatoes. This recipe is a nutritious and flavorful addition to your meal.

Total Prep Time:

30 minutes

Ingredients:

- 4 large tomatoes
- 1 cup quinoa, cooked
- Kale, finely chopped
- Red onion, finely diced
- Garlic, minced
- Feta cheese, crumbled
- Olive oil
- Lemon juice
- Salt and pepper to taste
- Fresh parsley for garnish

Instructions:

1. Preheat the oven to 375°F (190°C).

2. Cut the tops off the tomatoes and scoop out the seeds and pulp.
3. In a bowl, combine cooked quinoa, chopped kale, diced red onion, minced garlic, and crumbled feta cheese.
4. Drizzle with olive oil and lemon juice. Season with salt and pepper.
5. Stuff each tomato with the quinoa and kale mixture.
6. Place stuffed tomatoes in a baking dish and bake for 20-25 minutes.
7. Garnish with fresh parsley before serving.

Nutritional Information:

(Per serving)

- Calories: 250
- Protein: 10g
- Fat: 8g
- Carbohydrates: 35g
- Fiber: 5g

Mediterranean Couscous Salad

Intro:

Mediterranean Couscous Salad is a refreshing and vibrant dish inspired by the flavors of the Mediterranean. With fluffy couscous, colorful vegetables, olives, and feta cheese, this salad is a delightful addition to any meal or a perfect standalone dish.

Total Prep Time:

20 minutes

Ingredients:

- 1 cup couscous, cooked
- Cherry tomatoes, halved
- Cucumber, diced

- Kalamata olives, pitted and sliced
- Red onion, finely chopped
- Feta cheese, crumbled
- Fresh parsley, chopped
- Olive oil
- Lemon juice
- Dried oregano
- Salt and pepper to taste

Instructions:

1. In a large bowl, fluff cooked couscous with a fork.
2. Add cherry tomatoes, diced cucumber, sliced Kalamata olives, chopped red onion, and crumbled feta cheese.
3. Drizzle with olive oil and lemon juice.
4. Sprinkle dried oregano, salt, and pepper to taste.
5. Toss the salad gently to combine all ingredients.
6. Garnish with fresh parsley before serving.

Nutritional Information:

(Per serving)

- Calories: 280
- Protein: 8g
- Fat: 12g
- Carbohydrates: 35g
- Fiber: 5g

Stir-Fried Tofu with Broccoli and Brown Rice

Intro:

Stir-Fried Tofu with Broccoli and Brown Rice is a quick and nutritious dish that combines protein-packed tofu, vibrant broccoli, and wholesome brown rice. This stir-fry is both satisfying and flavorful, making it a perfect weeknight dinner.

Total Prep Time:

25 minutes

Ingredients:

- 1 block firm tofu, cubed
- Broccoli florets
- Carrots, julienned
- Bell peppers, sliced
- Brown rice, cooked
- Soy sauce
- Sesame oil
- Garlic, minced
- Ginger, grated
- Red pepper flakes (optional)
- Green onions for garnish

Instructions:

1. In a wok or skillet, heat sesame oil over medium-high heat.
2. Add cubed tofu and stir-fry until golden.
3. Add broccoli, julienned carrots, and sliced bell peppers.
4. Stir in minced garlic and grated ginger.
5. Drizzle with soy sauce and add red pepper flakes if desired.
6. Continue to stir-fry until vegetables are crisp-tender.
7. Serve over cooked brown rice.
8. Garnish with sliced green onions.

Nutritional Information:

(Per serving)

- Calories: 320
- Protein: 15g
- Fat: 12g
- Carbohydrates: 40g
- Fiber: 8g

Zucchini Noodles with Pesto and Cherry Tomatoes

Intro:

Zucchini Noodles with Pesto and Cherry Tomatoes offer a low-carb and flavorful twist on traditional pasta. Spiralized zucchini noodles are tossed with homemade pesto and juicy cherry tomatoes, creating a light and satisfying dish.

Total Prep Time:

15 minutes

Ingredients:

- Zucchini, spiralized into noodles
- Cherry tomatoes, halved
- Fresh basil leaves
- Parmesan cheese, grated
- Pine nuts
- Garlic, minced
- Olive oil
- Lemon juice
- Salt and pepper to taste

Instructions:

1. In a pan, lightly sauté spiralized zucchini noodles until just tender.

2. In a food processor, combine fresh basil, grated Parmesan cheese, pine nuts, minced garlic, and olive oil. Blend until smooth.
3. Toss the zucchini noodles with the homemade pesto.
4. Add cherry tomatoes and drizzle with lemon juice.
5. Season with salt and pepper to taste.
6. Serve these Zucchini Noodles with Pesto and Cherry Tomatoes as a refreshing and low-carb meal.

Nutritional Information:
(Per serving)
- Calories: 220
- Protein: 8g
- Fat: 18g
- Carbohydrates: 10g
- Fiber: 4g

Chicken Caesar Salad with Whole Grain Croutons

Intro:
Chicken Caesar Salad with Whole Grain Croutons is a classic and satisfying dish that combines crisp romaine lettuce, grilled chicken, whole grain croutons, and a creamy Caesar dressing. This salad is a balanced and delicious option for a light lunch or dinner.

Total Prep Time:
25 minutes

Ingredients:
- 2 boneless, skinless chicken breasts
- Romaine lettuce, chopped
- Whole grain bread, cut into cubes for croutons

- Olive oil
- Parmesan cheese, shaved
- Caesar dressing (store-bought or homemade)
- Lemon wedges for garnish
- Salt and pepper to taste

Instructions:
1. Preheat a grill or grill pan over medium-high heat.
2. Season chicken breasts with salt and pepper and grill until cooked through.
3. In a separate pan, toss cubed whole grain bread with olive oil and toast until golden to make croutons.
4. Slice grilled chicken into strips.
5. In a large bowl, combine chopped romaine lettuce, grilled chicken strips, whole grain croutons, and shaved Parmesan cheese.
6. Drizzle with Caesar dressing and toss gently to coat.
7. Garnish with lemon wedges before serving.

Nutritional Information:
(Per serving)
- Calories: 380
- Protein: 30g
- Fat: 20g
- Carbohydrates: 20g
- Fiber: 5g

Vegetable and Barley Soup

Intro:
Vegetable and Barley Soup is a hearty and nutritious soup that combines the wholesome goodness of barley with an array of colorful vegetables. This comforting soup is perfect

for a cozy meal and provides a satisfying combination of
flavors and textures.

Total Prep Time:
45 minutes

Ingredients:
- 1 cup pearl barley, rinsed
- Carrots, diced
- Celery, chopped
- Onion, finely chopped
- Garlic, minced
- Zucchini, diced
- Canned diced tomatoes
- Vegetable broth
- Bay leaves
- Thyme, dried or fresh
- Salt and pepper to taste
- Fresh parsley for garnish

Instructions:
1. In a large pot, combine rinsed pearl barley, diced carrots, chopped celery, finely chopped onion, and minced garlic.
2. Add diced zucchini, canned diced tomatoes, vegetable broth, bay leaves, and thyme.
3. Bring the soup to a boil, then reduce heat and simmer for 30-35 minutes or until barley is tender.
4. Season with salt and pepper to taste.
5. Remove bay leaves before serving.
6. Garnish with fresh parsley.

Nutritional Information:
(Per serving)
- Calories: 280

- Protein: 8g
- Fat: 2g
- Carbohydrates: 60g
- Fiber: 12g

Baked Cod with Lemon and Herbs

Intro:
Baked Cod with Lemon and Herbs is a light and flavorful dish that showcases the delicate taste of cod. The combination of zesty lemon and aromatic herbs enhances the natural richness of the fish. This recipe is perfect for a quick and healthy dinner.

Total Prep Time:
25 minutes

Ingredients:
- Cod fillets
- Lemon, sliced
- Fresh parsley, chopped
- Fresh dill, chopped
- Olive oil
- Garlic, minced
- Salt and pepper to taste

Instructions:
1. Preheat the oven to 375°F (190°C).
2. Place cod fillets on a baking sheet.
3. Drizzle with olive oil and sprinkle minced garlic, chopped parsley, and dill over the fillets.
4. Arrange lemon slices on top.
5. Bake for 15-20 minutes or until the cod is cooked through.
6. Season with salt and pepper to taste.

7. Serve this Baked Cod with Lemon and Herbs with your favorite side dishes.

Nutritional Information:
(Per serving)
- Calories: 180
- Protein: 25g
- Fat: 8g
- Carbohydrates: 2g
- Fiber: 1g

Roasted Vegetable and Chickpea Bowl

Intro:
Roasted Vegetable and Chickpea Bowl is a nutritious and satisfying meal that combines colorful roasted vegetables with protein-packed chickpeas. The variety of textures and flavors make this bowl a delightful and wholesome choice for lunch or dinner.

Total Prep Time:
30 minutes

Ingredients:
- Assorted vegetables (bell peppers, zucchini, cherry tomatoes, etc.)
- Chickpeas, drained and rinsed
- Olive oil
- Paprika, cumin, and garlic powder
- Salt and pepper to taste
- Quinoa or brown rice for serving
- Fresh herbs for garnish

Instructions:
1. Preheat the oven to 400°F (200°C).

2. Toss assorted vegetables and chickpeas with olive oil, paprika, cumin, garlic powder, salt, and pepper.
3. Spread the mixture on a baking sheet and roast for 20-25 minutes, or until vegetables are tender.
4. Serve over quinoa or brown rice.
5. Garnish with fresh herbs before serving.

Nutritional Information:
(Per serving)
- Calories: 350
- Protein: 12g
- Fat: 10g
- Carbohydrates: 55g
- Fiber: 12g

Turkey Meatballs with Zucchini Noodles

Intro:
Turkey Meatballs with Zucchini Noodles is a lighter take on the classic spaghetti and meatballs. Tender turkey meatballs are paired with spiralized zucchini noodles and a flavorful tomato sauce, creating a low-carb and delicious alternative.

Total Prep Time:
40 minutes

Ingredients:
- Ground turkey
- Bread crumbs
- Egg
- Garlic, minced
- Italian seasoning
- Salt and pepper to taste
- Zucchini, spiralized

- Tomato sauce
- Parmesan cheese for garnish

Instructions:
1. Preheat the oven to 375°F (190°C).
2. In a bowl, combine ground turkey, bread crumbs, egg, minced garlic, Italian seasoning, salt, and pepper. Form into meatballs.
3. Bake meatballs for 20-25 minutes or until cooked through.
4. In a pan, heat tomato sauce and add the cooked meatballs.
5. Spiralize zucchini and sauté in a separate pan until just tender.
6. Serve meatballs over zucchini noodles.
7. Garnish with Parmesan cheese.

Nutritional Information:
(Per serving)
- Calories: 280
- Protein: 25g
- Fat: 12g
- Carbohydrates: 20g
- Fiber: 5g

Cauliflower Fried Rice with Shrimp

Intro:
Cauliflower Fried Rice with Shrimp is a low-carb and flavorful alternative to traditional fried rice. Cauliflower rice is stir-fried with shrimp, vegetables, and savory seasonings, creating a satisfying and nutritious dish.

Total Prep Time:
25 minutes

Ingredients:

- Cauliflower, riced
- Shrimp, peeled and deveined
- Mixed vegetables (peas, carrots, corn, etc.)
- Soy sauce
- Sesame oil
- Garlic, minced
- Ginger, grated
- Green onions, sliced
- Eggs, beaten (optional)

Instructions:

1. In a large pan, heat sesame oil and sauté minced garlic and grated ginger.
2. Add shrimp and cook until pink.
3. Add mixed vegetables and cook until tender.
4. Push ingredients to the side and scramble beaten eggs if using.
5. Stir in cauliflower rice and soy sauce.
6. Cook until cauliflower is tender.
7. Garnish with sliced green onions before serving.

Nutritional Information:

(Per serving)

- Calories: 250
- Protein: 20g
- Fat: 10g
- Carbohydrates: 15g
- Fiber: 5g

Grilled Eggplant and Tomato Stack

Intro:

Grilled Eggplant and Tomato Stack is a visually appealing and delicious dish that combines the smokiness of grilled eggplant with the freshness of ripe tomatoes and mozzarella. This simple yet elegant recipe makes for a delightful appetizer or side dish.

Total Prep Time:

30 minutes

Ingredients:

- Eggplant, sliced
- Tomatoes, sliced
- Fresh mozzarella, sliced
- Balsamic glaze
- Olive oil
- Fresh basil leaves
- Salt and pepper to taste

Instructions:

1. Preheat the grill or grill pan.
2. Brush eggplant slices with olive oil and season with salt and pepper.
3. Grill eggplant until tender and grill marks appear.
4. Assemble stacks by layering grilled eggplant, sliced tomatoes, and fresh mozzarella.
5. Drizzle with balsamic glaze.
6. Garnish with fresh basil leaves before serving.

Nutritional Information:

(Per serving)

- Calories: 180
- Protein: 10g
- Fat: 12g

- Carbohydrates: 10g
- Fiber: 4g

Quinoa and Spinach Stuffed Mushrooms

Intro:
Quinoa and Spinach Stuffed Mushrooms are a tasty and nutritious appetizer or side dish. The earthy flavor of mushrooms pairs perfectly with the savory quinoa and vibrant spinach, creating a delightful bite-sized treat.

Total Prep Time:
30 minutes

Ingredients:
- Large mushrooms, cleaned and stems removed
- Quinoa, cooked
- Baby spinach, chopped
- Red onion, finely diced
- Garlic, minced
- Feta cheese, crumbled
- Olive oil
- Lemon juice
- Salt and pepper to taste
- Fresh parsley for garnish

Instructions:
1. Preheat the oven to 375°F (190°C).
2. In a pan, sauté red onion and minced garlic in olive oil until softened.
3. Add chopped baby spinach and cook until wilted.
4. In a bowl, combine cooked quinoa, sautéed spinach mixture, crumbled feta, and lemon juice. Season with salt and pepper.
5. Stuff mushrooms with the quinoa mixture.

6. Place stuffed mushrooms on a baking sheet and bake for 15-20 minutes.
7. Garnish with fresh parsley before serving.

Nutritional Information:

(Per serving)
- Calories: 120
- Protein: 5g
- Fat: 6g
- Carbohydrates: 15g
- Fiber: 3g

Chicken and Broccoli Stir-Fry

Intro:

Chicken and Broccoli Stir-Fry is a quick and flavorful dish that combines tender pieces of chicken with crisp broccoli in a savory stir-fry sauce. This recipe is perfect for a busy weeknight dinner, providing a balance of protein and vegetables.

Total Prep Time:

20 minutes

Ingredients:

- Chicken breast, thinly sliced
- Broccoli florets
- Soy sauce
- Oyster sauce
- Garlic, minced
- Ginger, grated
- Sesame oil
- Cornstarch
- Olive oil
- Rice or noodles for serving

Instructions:

1. In a bowl, mix soy sauce, oyster sauce, minced garlic, grated ginger, sesame oil, and cornstarch to create the sauce.
2. Heat olive oil in a wok or skillet over high heat.
3. Add sliced chicken and stir-fry until browned and cooked through.
4. Add broccoli florets and continue stir-frying until tender-crisp.
5. Pour the sauce over the chicken and broccoli, stirring to coat evenly.
6. Cook for an additional 2-3 minutes until the sauce thickens.
7. Serve over rice or noodles.

Nutritional Information:

(Per serving)

- Calories: 300
- Protein: 25g
- Fat: 12g
- Carbohydrates: 20g
- Fiber: 4g

Sweet Potato and Lentil Curry

Intro:

Sweet Potato and Lentil Curry is a hearty and flavorful vegetarian dish that combines the natural sweetness of sweet potatoes with the protein-rich goodness of lentils. This curry is a comforting option for a satisfying and nutritious meal.

Total Prep Time:

45 minutes

Ingredients:

- Sweet potatoes, peeled and diced
- Lentils, rinsed
- Onion, finely chopped
- Garlic, minced
- Ginger, grated
- Curry powder
- Coconut milk
- Vegetable broth
- Tomatoes, diced
- Spinach leaves
- Olive oil
- Salt and pepper to taste
- Cilantro for garnish
- Cooked rice for serving

Instructions:

1. In a pot, sauté chopped onion, minced garlic, and grated ginger in olive oil until softened.
2. Add curry powder and stir to coat the onions.
3. Add diced sweet potatoes, rinsed lentils, coconut milk, vegetable broth, and diced tomatoes.
4. Simmer until sweet potatoes and lentils are tender.
5. Stir in fresh spinach leaves and cook until wilted.
6. Season with salt and pepper to taste.
7. Serve this Sweet Potato and Lentil Curry over cooked rice.
8. Garnish with cilantro.

Nutritional Information:

(Per serving)

- Calories: 320
- Protein: 15g
- Fat: 8g

- Carbohydrates: 50g
- Fiber: 10g

Baked Salmon with Dill and Garlic

Intro:
Baked Salmon with Dill and Garlic is a simple and elegant dish that highlights the natural flavors of salmon. The combination of fresh dill and garlic enhances the richness of the salmon, creating a delicious and healthy main course.

Total Prep Time:
25 minutes

Ingredients:
- Salmon fillets
- Fresh dill, chopped
- Garlic, minced
- Lemon juice
- Olive oil
- Salt and pepper to taste

Instructions:
1. Preheat the oven to 375°F (190°C).
2. Place salmon fillets on a baking sheet.
3. In a bowl, mix chopped fresh dill, minced garlic, lemon juice, and olive oil.
4. Spread the dill and garlic mixture over the salmon fillets.
5. Season with salt and pepper to taste.
6. Bake for 15-20 minutes or until the salmon is cooked through.
7. Serve this Baked Salmon with Dill and Garlic with your favorite side dishes.

Nutritional Information:
(Per serving)

- Calories: 250
- Protein: 25g
- Fat: 15g
- Carbohydrates: 1g
- Fiber: 0g

Spaghetti Squash with Tomato and Basil Sauce

Intro:

Spaghetti Squash with Tomato and Basil Sauce is a low-carb alternative to traditional pasta dishes. The strands of spaghetti squash are paired with a flavorful tomato and basil sauce, creating a satisfying and lighter option for pasta lovers.

Total Prep Time:

40 minutes

Ingredients:

- Spaghetti squash, halved and seeds removed
- Tomatoes, diced
- Fresh basil, chopped
- Garlic, minced
- Olive oil
- Red pepper flakes (optional)
- Salt and pepper to taste
- Parmesan cheese for garnish

Instructions:

1. Preheat the oven to 375°F (190°C).

2. Place spaghetti squash halves, cut side down, on a baking sheet. Roast for 30-35 minutes or until tender.
3. In a pan, sauté minced garlic in olive oil until fragrant.
4. Add diced tomatoes and cook until they release their juices.
5. Stir in fresh basil, red pepper flakes if using, salt, and pepper.
6. Use a fork to scrape the strands of cooked spaghetti squash.
7. Toss the spaghetti squash with the tomato and basil sauce.
8. Garnish with Parmesan cheese before serving.

Nutritional Information:
(Per serving)
- Calories: 150
- Protein: 3g
- Fat: 8g
- Carbohydrates: 20g
- Fiber: 4g

Turkey and Vegetable Skewers

Intro:
Turkey and Vegetable Skewers are a flavorful and healthy option for grilling enthusiasts. The combination of marinated turkey, colorful vegetables, and a hint of smokiness from the grill make these skewers a perfect addition to any barbecue.

Total Prep Time:
30 minutes

Ingredients:

- Turkey breast, cut into cubes
- Bell peppers, cut into chunks
- Red onion, cut into wedges
- Cherry tomatoes
- Zucchini, sliced
- Olive oil
- Lemon juice
- Garlic, minced
- Italian seasoning
- Salt and pepper to taste

Instructions:

1. In a bowl, whisk together olive oil, lemon juice, minced garlic, Italian seasoning, salt, and pepper to create the marinade.
2. Thread marinated turkey cubes, bell pepper chunks, red onion wedges, cherry tomatoes, and zucchini slices onto skewers.
3. Preheat the grill to medium-high heat.
4. Grill skewers for 10-15 minutes, turning occasionally, until turkey is cooked through and vegetables are tender.
5. Serve these Turkey and Vegetable Skewers with your favorite side dishes.

Nutritional Information:

(Per serving)

- Calories: 220
- Protein: 25g
- Fat: 10g
- Carbohydrates: 10g
- Fiber: 2g

Quinoa-stuffed Bell Peppers with Ground Turkey

Intro:

Quinoa-stuffed Bell Peppers with Ground Turkey are a wholesome and colorful dish that combines the nutty flavor of quinoa with lean ground turkey, creating a protein-packed and satisfying meal. These stuffed peppers are baked to perfection, making them a nutritious addition to your dinner table.

Total Prep Time:

40 minutes

Ingredients:

- Bell peppers, halved and seeds removed
- Quinoa, cooked
- Ground turkey
- Onion, finely diced
- Garlic, minced
- Tomato sauce
- Black beans, drained and rinsed
- Corn kernels
- Cumin, paprika, and chili powder
- Salt and pepper to taste
- Shredded cheese for topping

Instructions:

1. Preheat the oven to 375°F (190°C).
2. In a pan, cook ground turkey until browned.
3. Add finely diced onion and minced garlic, sautéing until softened.
4. Stir in cooked quinoa, tomato sauce, black beans, corn, cumin, paprika, chili powder, salt, and pepper.

5. Fill bell pepper halves with the quinoa and turkey mixture.
6. Top each stuffed pepper with shredded cheese.
7. Bake for 20-25 minutes or until the peppers are tender.
8. Serve these Quinoa-stuffed Bell Peppers with your favorite toppings.

Nutritional Information:
(Per serving)
- Calories: 280
- Protein: 20g
- Fat: 10g
- Carbohydrates: 30g
- Fiber: 6g

Black Bean and Corn Quesadillas

Intro:
Black Bean and Corn Quesadillas are a quick and satisfying option for a flavorful lunch or dinner. The combination of black beans, corn, melted cheese, and warm tortillas creates a delicious and easy-to-make meal.

Total Prep Time:
20 minutes

Ingredients:
- Flour tortillas
- Black beans, cooked and mashed
- Corn kernels
- Red onion, finely diced
- Jalapeño, sliced (optional)
- Shredded cheese (cheddar or Mexican blend)
- Cumin and chili powder

- Olive oil for cooking
- Guacamole and salsa for serving

Instructions:
1. In a bowl, mix mashed black beans, corn kernels, diced red onion, sliced jalapeño (if using), cumin, and chili powder.
2. Place a spoonful of the black bean mixture on one half of a tortilla.
3. Sprinkle shredded cheese over the bean mixture.
4. Fold the tortilla in half to create a quesadilla.
5. Heat olive oil in a pan over medium heat.
6. Cook the quesadillas for 2-3 minutes on each side, until the tortillas are golden and the cheese is melted.
7. Serve these Black Bean and Corn Quesadillas with guacamole and salsa.

Nutritional Information:
(Per serving)
- Calories: 300
- Protein: 12g
- Fat: 10g
- Carbohydrates: 40g
- Fiber: 6g

Lemon Garlic Chicken with Roasted Brussels Sprouts

Intro:
Lemon Garlic Chicken with Roasted Brussels Sprouts is a flavorful and wholesome dish that brings together tender chicken breasts with zesty lemon and aromatic garlic. The addition of roasted Brussels sprouts completes the meal, offering a balance of protein and vegetables.

Total Prep Time:
40 minutes

Ingredients:
- Chicken breasts
- Lemon, sliced
- Garlic, minced
- Olive oil
- Thyme, dried or fresh
- Brussels sprouts, halved
- Salt and pepper to taste

Instructions:
1. Preheat the oven to 400°F (200°C).
2. Place chicken breasts in a baking dish.
3. Arrange lemon slices over the chicken and sprinkle minced garlic and thyme.
4. Drizzle with olive oil and season with salt and pepper.
5. In a separate baking dish, toss halved Brussels sprouts with olive oil, salt, and pepper.
6. Bake both the chicken and Brussels sprouts for 25-30 minutes or until the chicken is cooked through and Brussels sprouts are golden and crispy.
7. Serve this Lemon Garlic Chicken with Roasted Brussels Sprouts with your favorite side dishes.

Nutritional Information:
(Per serving)
- Calories: 320
- Protein: 30g
- Fat: 12g
- Carbohydrates: 20g
- Fiber: 8g

Lentil and Vegetable Soup

Intro:

Lentil and Vegetable Soup is a comforting and nutritious dish that combines the earthy flavor of brown lentils with a medley of colorful vegetables. This hearty soup is perfect for a wholesome and satisfying meal.

Total Prep Time:

45 minutes

Ingredients:
- Brown lentils, rinsed
- Carrots, diced
- Celery, chopped
- Onion, finely chopped
- Garlic, minced
- Tomatoes, diced
- Vegetable broth
- Bay leaves
- Thyme, dried or fresh
- Spinach leaves
- Olive oil
- Salt and pepper to taste
- Fresh parsley for garnish

Instructions:
1. In a large pot, sauté onions and garlic in olive oil until softened.
2. Add diced carrots, chopped celery, and tomatoes. Cook until vegetables are tender.
3. Pour in vegetable broth, add bay leaves and thyme, and bring to a simmer.
4. Stir in brown lentils and cook until lentils are tender.

5. Add spinach leaves and cook until wilted.
6. Season with salt and pepper to taste.
7. Garnish with fresh parsley before serving.

Nutritional Information:
(Per serving)
- Calories: 250
- Protein: 12g
- Fat: 5g
- Carbohydrates: 40g
- Fiber: 12g

Baked Teriyaki Tofu with Steamed Brown Rice

Intro:
Baked Teriyaki Tofu with Steamed Brown Rice is a flavorful and plant-based dish that brings together the savory goodness of teriyaki-marinated tofu with wholesome brown rice. This recipe is a delicious and satisfying option for those looking to incorporate more plant-based meals into their diet.

Total Prep Time:
50 minutes

Ingredients:
- Firm tofu, pressed and cubed
- Teriyaki sauce (store-bought or homemade)
- Brown rice, cooked
- Broccoli florets
- Sesame seeds for garnish
- Green onions, sliced for garnish

Instructions:

1. Preheat the oven to 375°F (190°C).
2. Marinate cubed tofu in teriyaki sauce for at least 30 minutes.
3. Place marinated tofu on a baking sheet and bake for 25-30 minutes, turning halfway through, until golden and crispy.
4. Steam broccoli florets until tender-crisp.
5. Serve baked teriyaki tofu over steamed brown rice, garnished with sesame seeds and sliced green onions.

Nutritional Information:

(Per serving)

- Calories: 320
- Protein: 15g
- Fat: 12g
- Carbohydrates: 40g
- Fiber: 6g

Greek-Style Baked Chicken with Olives and Tomatoes

Intro:

Greek-Style Baked Chicken with Olives and Tomatoes is a Mediterranean-inspired dish that combines juicy chicken with the briny flavor of olives and the sweetness of roasted tomatoes. This flavorful recipe is a delightful addition to your dinner table.

Total Prep Time:

55 minutes

Ingredients:

- Chicken thighs, bone-in and skin-on
- Kalamata olives, pitted

- Cherry tomatoes
- Red onion, sliced
- Garlic, minced
- Olive oil
- Lemon juice
- Oregano, dried or fresh
- Salt and pepper to taste
- Feta cheese for garnish
- Fresh parsley for garnish

Instructions:
1. Preheat the oven to 400°F (200°C).
2. In a bowl, toss chicken thighs, olives, cherry tomatoes, sliced red onion, and minced garlic with olive oil, lemon juice, oregano, salt, and pepper.
3. Arrange the mixture in a baking dish.
4. Bake for 35-40 minutes or until the chicken is cooked through and the skin is crispy.
5. Garnish with crumbled feta cheese and fresh parsley before serving.

Nutritional Information:
(Per serving)
- Calories: 380
- Protein: 25g
- Fat: 22g
- Carbohydrates: 15g
- Fiber: 4g

Vegetable and Tofu Stir-Fry with Brown Rice

Intro:

Vegetable and Tofu Stir-Fry with Brown Rice is a colorful and nutrient-packed dish that combines a variety of crisp vegetables and protein-rich tofu. The light and flavorful stir-fry sauce brings everything together for a delicious and wholesome meal.

Total Prep Time:

30 minutes

Ingredients:
- Firm tofu, pressed and cubed
- Broccoli florets
- Bell peppers, sliced
- Carrots, julienned
- Snow peas
- Brown rice, cooked
- Sesame oil
- Soy sauce
- Rice vinegar
- Garlic, minced
- Ginger, grated
- Red pepper flakes (optional)
- Green onions, sliced for garnish

Instructions:
1. In a wok or large pan, heat sesame oil over medium-high heat.
2. Add cubed tofu and stir-fry until golden and crispy.
3. Add broccoli florets, sliced bell peppers, julienned carrots, and snow peas. Stir-fry until vegetables are tender-crisp.

4. In a small bowl, whisk together soy sauce, rice vinegar, minced garlic, grated ginger, and red pepper flakes if using.
5. Pour the sauce over the tofu and vegetables, tossing to coat evenly.
6. Serve the stir-fry over cooked brown rice, garnished with sliced green onions.

Nutritional Information:

(Per serving)

- Calories: 320
- Protein: 15g
- Fat: 12g
- Carbohydrates: 40g
- Fiber: 6g

Grilled Swordfish with Mango Salsa

Intro:

Grilled Swordfish with Mango Salsa is a vibrant and tropical dish that pairs succulent grilled swordfish with a refreshing mango salsa. This recipe is a delightful combination of flavors and textures, making it a perfect choice for a light and flavorful dinner.

Total Prep Time:

40 minutes

Ingredients:

- Swordfish steaks
- Mango, diced
- Red onion, finely chopped
- Jalapeño, finely diced
- Cilantro, chopped
- Lime juice

- Olive oil
- Salt and pepper to taste

Instructions:
1. Preheat the grill to medium-high heat.
2. Season swordfish steaks with olive oil, salt, and pepper.
3. Grill swordfish for 4-5 minutes per side or until cooked through.
4. In a bowl, combine diced mango, finely chopped red onion, diced jalapeño, chopped cilantro, lime juice, and a pinch of salt.
5. Spoon mango salsa over grilled swordfish before serving.

Nutritional Information:
(Per serving)
- Calories: 280
- Protein: 25g
- Fat: 15g
- Carbohydrates: 15g
- Fiber: 3g

Zucchini and Tomato Gratin

Intro:
Zucchini and Tomato Gratin is a savory and cheesy casserole that showcases the flavors of fresh zucchini and ripe tomatoes. This gratin is a delightful side dish or a light vegetarian main course.

Total Prep Time:
50 minutes

Ingredients:
- Zucchini, thinly sliced

- Tomatoes, thinly sliced
- Onion, thinly sliced
- Garlic, minced
- Parmesan cheese, grated
- Mozzarella cheese, shredded
- Olive oil
- Fresh basil, chopped
- Salt and pepper to taste

Instructions:
1. Preheat the oven to 375°F (190°C).
2. In a skillet, sauté thinly sliced zucchini, tomatoes, and onions in olive oil until slightly softened.
3. Add minced garlic and cook for an additional minute.
4. In a greased baking dish, layer the sautéed vegetables.
5. Sprinkle grated Parmesan and shredded mozzarella over the vegetables.
6. Repeat the layers, finishing with a layer of cheese on top.
7. Bake for 25-30 minutes or until the cheese is golden and bubbly.
8. Garnish with chopped fresh basil before serving.

Nutritional Information:
(Per serving)
- Calories: 200
- Protein: 10g
- Fat: 12g
- Carbohydrates: 15g
- Fiber: 5g

Quinoa and Black Bean Casserole

Intro:
Quinoa and Black Bean Casserole is a protein-packed and flavorful dish that combines the nuttiness of quinoa with the richness of black beans. This casserole is a wholesome and satisfying option for a vegetarian or vegan meal.

Total Prep Time:
45 minutes

Ingredients:
- Quinoa, cooked
- Black beans, cooked and drained
- Corn kernels
- Bell peppers, diced
- Onion, finely chopped
- Garlic, minced
- Tomato sauce
- Cumin, chili powder, and paprika
- Shredded cheese (cheddar or Mexican blend)
- Fresh cilantro for garnish
- Avocado slices for serving

Instructions:
1. Preheat the oven to 375°F (190°C).
2. In a large bowl, mix cooked quinoa, black beans, corn kernels, diced bell peppers, chopped onion, minced garlic, tomato sauce, cumin, chili powder, and paprika.
3. Transfer the mixture to a greased baking dish.
4. Sprinkle shredded cheese over the top.
5. Bake for 25-30 minutes or until the casserole is heated through and the cheese is melted.

6. Garnish with fresh cilantro and serve with avocado slices.

Nutritional Information:
(Per serving)
- Calories: 320
- Protein: 15g
- Fat: 12g
- Carbohydrates: 40g
- Fiber: 8g

Chicken and Vegetable Kebabs

Intro:
Chicken and Vegetable Kebabs are a delightful and customizable grilling option that brings together marinated chicken with a variety of colorful vegetables. These kebabs are perfect for outdoor gatherings and provide a balanced combination of protein and veggies.

Total Prep Time:
40 minutes

Ingredients:
- Chicken breast, cut into cubes
- Bell peppers, cut into chunks
- Red onion, cut into wedges
- Cherry tomatoes
- Zucchini, sliced
- Olive oil
- Lemon juice
- Garlic, minced
- Italian seasoning
- Salt and pepper to taste

Instructions:

1. In a bowl, whisk together olive oil, lemon juice, minced garlic, Italian seasoning, salt, and pepper to create the marinade.
2. Thread marinated chicken cubes, bell pepper chunks, red onion wedges, cherry tomatoes, and zucchini slices onto skewers.
3. Preheat the grill to medium-high heat.
4. Grill kebabs for 10-15 minutes, turning occasionally, until chicken is cooked through and vegetables are tender.
5. Serve these Chicken and Vegetable Kebabs with your favorite side dishes.

Nutritional Information:
(Per serving)

- Calories: 220
- Protein: 25g
- Fat: 10g
- Carbohydrates: 10g
- Fiber: 2g

Shrimp and Quinoa Paella

Intro:
Shrimp and Quinoa Paella is a lighter and quicker version of the traditional Spanish dish, using protein-packed quinoa instead of rice. This recipe combines the flavors of saffron, garlic, and paprika with succulent shrimp for a delightful and nutritious paella.

Total Prep Time:
40 minutes

Ingredients:

- Shrimp, peeled and deveined

- Quinoa, rinsed
- Bell peppers, diced
- Onion, finely chopped
- Tomatoes, diced
- Garlic, minced
- Saffron threads
- Smoked paprika
- Vegetable broth
- Olive oil
- Lemon wedges for serving
- Fresh parsley for garnish

Instructions:
1. In a bowl, soak saffron threads in a little warm water.
2. In a paella pan or large skillet, sauté chopped onion and minced garlic in olive oil until softened.
3. Add diced bell peppers and tomatoes, cooking until softened.
4. Stir in smoked paprika and rinsed quinoa, coating the grains in the flavorful mixture.
5. Pour in vegetable broth and add saffron-infused water. Bring to a simmer.
6. Arrange shrimp on top of the quinoa mixture and cook until shrimp are pink and opaque.
7. Garnish with fresh parsley and serve with lemon wedges.

Nutritional Information:
(Per serving)
- Calories: 320
- Protein: 25g
- Fat: 10g
- Carbohydrates: 30g

- Fiber: 5g

Stuffed Acorn Squash with Wild Rice

Intro:
Stuffed Acorn Squash with Wild Rice is a wholesome and flavorful dish that brings together the nutty taste of wild rice with the natural sweetness of acorn squash. This recipe is a perfect balance of textures and tastes, making it an excellent option for a comforting meal.

Total Prep Time:
50 minutes

Ingredients:
- Acorn squash, halved and seeds removed
- Wild rice, cooked
- Pecans, chopped
- Cranberries, dried
- Onion, finely chopped
- Celery, diced
- Garlic, minced
- Vegetable broth
- Sage, dried or fresh
- Olive oil
- Salt and pepper to taste

Instructions:
1. Preheat the oven to 375°F (190°C).
2. Place acorn squash halves, cut side down, on a baking sheet. Roast for 25-30 minutes or until tender.
3. In a pan, sauté chopped onion, diced celery, and minced garlic in olive oil until softened.

4. Add cooked wild rice, chopped pecans, dried cranberries, vegetable broth, and sage. Cook until heated through.
5. Season with salt and pepper to taste.
6. Stuff the roasted acorn squash halves with the wild rice mixture.
7. Bake for an additional 15 minutes.
8. Serve these Stuffed Acorn Squash with a drizzle of olive oil.

Nutritional Information:
(Per serving)
- Calories: 280
- Protein: 6g
- Fat: 10g
- Carbohydrates: 45g
- Fiber: 7g

Eggplant Lasagna with Whole Wheat Noodles

Intro:
Eggplant Lasagna with Whole Wheat Noodles is a healthier twist on the classic Italian dish. Instead of traditional pasta, this recipe uses whole wheat noodles, and layers of roasted eggplant and a rich tomato sauce, creating a flavorful and satisfying lasagna.

Total Prep Time:
60 minutes

Ingredients:
- Eggplant, thinly sliced
- Whole wheat lasagna noodles, cooked
- Ricotta cheese
- Spinach leaves

- Mozzarella cheese, shredded
- Parmesan cheese, grated
- Tomato sauce
- Garlic, minced
- Basil, dried or fresh
- Olive oil
- Salt and pepper to taste

Instructions:
1. Preheat the oven to 375°F (190°C).
2. Brush eggplant slices with olive oil and roast in the oven until tender.
3. In a bowl, mix ricotta cheese with minced garlic, dried basil, salt, and pepper.
4. In a baking dish, layer whole wheat lasagna noodles, roasted eggplant slices, spinach leaves, ricotta mixture, and shredded mozzarella.
5. Repeat the layers, finishing with a layer of tomato sauce on top.
6. Sprinkle grated Parmesan cheese over the lasagna.
7. Bake for 30-35 minutes or until the cheese is bubbly and golden.
8. Let it rest for a few minutes before serving.

Nutritional Information:
(Per serving)
- Calories: 350
- Protein: 18g
- Fat: 15g
- Carbohydrates: 40g
- Fiber: 7g

www.ingramcontent.com/pod-product-compliance
Lightning Source LLC
Chambersburg PA
CBHW060945260726
48661CB00005B/1760